THE NEW WAY

TO TAKE CHARGE

OF YOUR

MEDICAL TREATMENT

THE NEW WAY

TO TAKE CHARGE

OF YOUR

MEDICAL TREATMENT

A PATIENT'S GUIDE

By
Barbara Hardt, CSW
and
Katharine R. Halkin

Madison Books
Lanham • New York • London

Published by Madison Books
4720 Boston Way
Lanham, Maryland 20706

3 Henrietta Street
London WC2E 8LU England

Distributed by National Book Network

The paper used in this publication meets minimum require-
ments of American National Standard for Information Sci-
ences — Permanence of Paper for Printed Library Materials,
ANSI Z39.48 — 1984.⊚™
Manufactured in the United States of America.

Library of Congress Cataloging-in-Publication Data

Hardt, Barbara
    The new way to take charge of your medical treat-
ment : a patient's guide / by Barbara Hardt and Katharine
R. Halkin.
        p. cm.
    Includes bibliographical references and index.
    1. Patients—Legal status, laws, etc.—United States
— Popular works. 2. Informed consent (Medical law)—
United State—Popular works. I. Halkin, Katharine R.
II. Title.
KD3823.Z9H37   1995
344.73'0412—dc20
[347.304412]

ISBN 1-56833-034-0 (pbk: alk.paper)

We dedicate this book to our children: David, Steven, Mark, Jennifer, Paul, Ken and Tim.

Their love, support and advocacy efforts on our behalf helped us to survive the many months of our hospitalizations.

CONTENTS

FOREWORD
by
Barry D. Rock, DSW

This book is above all about communication—
good communication in health care between the
patient and the provider of care. It is written as a
guide for patients but could be read to great benefit by health care professionals as well, since its
message is two-way communication. Communication in health care practice is not an extra or a
luxury, it is a necessity.

Hospitals and doctors, who often seem cold, de-
tached, and noncommunicative, rarely are that
way because of malice. They feel that their con-
tribution is fundamentally technical; their human-
ism is expressed by fully sharing their biomedical
knowledge, skill and technology. This narrow biomedical perspective inadvertently leaves out an
essential component—you, the patient, as a human being with very human fears and needs.
Truly excellent medical practice, in scientific
terms, requires that you be included as a person,
because you have many valuable things to contribute to the healing process.

This book is an excellent guide about how to contribute to your own healing and to the overall effectiveness of your medical care. It is written in an exceptionally clear and well organized way. It is, most importantly, highly supportive. The authors show you how to be more aggressive, yes, but in a very constructive way. The professionals who are caring for you should appreciate your efforts. In the long run, it will make life easier for them as well and improve the health care delivery system for us all.

Barry D. Rock, DSW, has 25 years experience in health care. He is the Director of the Department of Social Work Services of a large teaching medical center in the New York City area and is on the faculty of several universities. He has published 25 articles in professional journals.

PREFACE

We are two professionals in the field of human services with extensive training in advocacy. Nevertheless, in thinking back over the lengthy periods of hospitalization we have both endured, we realized that we had encountered many life-threatening or difficult situations that could have been avoided had we been aware of our rights as patients.

For Barbara, the first faint awareness of the concept of patient's rights came when she refused to take a particular test while in the hospital. A nurse informed her that, although she had the right to refuse, it was going to be noted on her chart. Intimidating? Yes; but illuminating as well. What she didn't know at the time was that the right to refuse tests is only one of many patient's rights. Katharine's initial introduction to patient's rights came near the end of her hospitalization, when a rehabilitation nurse explained that she did not have to take any medication she felt she did not need.

As a result of severe medical problems, each of us was in three separate hospitals. This means that we each received three copies of the

Patient's Bill of Rights as part of our packets of admissions materials. Yet, not once did anyone ever point out to either of us that a Bill of Rights was included, much less explain it.

We hope that this book will provide readers with the knowledge they need to ensure that they receive the best possible medical treatment.

The case histories in the book are all authentic, but we have changed some details to protect the identities of the patients. Nearly all incidents occurred in large, respected hospitals and medical centers in the metropolitan New York area.

ACKNOWLEDGMENTS

Many thanks to Marge Elias, RN, for introducing us and for intuitively knowing, even before we did, that we would write this book together.

Our gratitude also to Richard Thaler for his patience and skill in editing.

Finally, we wish to recognize the invaluable assistance we received from Alexandra Gekas, the Executive Director of the National Society for Patient Representation and Consumer Affairs of the American Hospital Association.

INTRODUCTION

A PATIENT'S BILL OF RIGHTS

Preamble

Gary's Story

Gary was rushed to the hospital emergency room after his mother found him lying on the floor, near death, as a result of a drug overdose. When Gary was no longer in immediate danger, he was transferred to the intensive care unit, in critical condition, so that he could be monitored closely. Several days later, when he began to feel better, he asked to go home. However, because of his attempted suicide, the hospital could not legally discharge him until he had been evaluated by a staff psychiatrist. During the evaluation, Gary admitted that he was still very depressed and was afraid that he might try to kill himself again. The doctor prescribed an anti-psychotic medication that appeared to lessen Gary's depression so that he could return home safely and continue his treatment as an out-patient.

After a period of time, Gary began having problems with his vision. He went to an ophthalmolo-
gist who referred him to a neurologist because his
vision was rapidly deteriorating. He was given a
battery of neurological tests, but none of these re-
vealed the cause. Eventually, the neurologist
traced Gary's loss of vision to the medicine the
psychiatrist had prescribed. Gary said he never
would have taken this medication, no matter how
depressed he was, had he been aware of this po-
tentially dangerous side effect. He sued the doctor for not making him aware this drug might
cause blindness, thus denying him HIS RIGHT
TO INFORMED CONSENT. Although the jury
awarded Gary several million dollars, the money
hardly compensates him for his permanent loss of
sight.

The tragic irony of Gary's story is that he had been given a copy of a document entitled A PATIENT'S BILL OF RIGHTS, along with many other official looking papers, soon after he was admitted to ICU, but he and his parents did not look at it because they were too upset by his suicide attempt. Instead, they just accepted, without question, whatever the hospital doctors told them. Implicit throughout the Bill of Rights is the concept of "informed consent." There is no way a patient can exercise his right to participate fully in his own treatment if he does not understand the various options available to him and all the ramifications thereof.

Gary happened to live in a state where hospitals are required by law to present a written statement of patients' rights upon admission. But, even in states that do not yet have this requirement, these rights exist.

Nevertheless, rights only have value when they are understood and enforced by those they are designed to protect.

Serious problems can arise in even the best medical facilities. Patients *must* exercise their rights and take responsibility for decisions regarding their care.

Ever since Hippocrates, patients have been intimidated by doctors and by hospital rules and regulations. Because doctors and hospitals exist only to make us well, we may feel presumptious and ungrateful if we question any of their services. Yet, we need to recognize that giving in to these feelings can be very damaging when our health is at stake. If we are to become enlightened health care consumers, we must be even more careful in purchasing medical services than we are when we buy houses, autos and appliances.

Fortunately, today many doctors and other health care professionals welcome the involvement of patients in their own medical treatment, so long as they act in a rational and organized manner.

This book will help your overcome your fears and insecurities about communicating with health care professionals by providing step-by-step instructions on how to guarantee your rights as a patient.

*Knowing your rights
can make it possible for
you to receive the best
quality health care.*

Patients' Rights
Questionnaire
(True or False)

1. In order to understand your rights as a hospital patient, your hospital must provide you with an interpreter if you are not conversant in English.   T_____ F_____

2. Your local hospital has the right to refuse treatment to AIDS patients.   T_____ F_____

3. You can be denied emergency care if you cannot pay for it.   T_____ F_____

4. Everyone involved in your care must tell you their name, position and function.
       T_____ F_____

5. If your doctor orders a particular diagnostic test, treatment or medication, you can't refuse to follow his directions.
       T_____ F_____

6. You cannot expect to be moved to a different room just because your roommate smokes.   T_____ F_____

7. If your medical situation is very grave, your doctor can use her discretion about how much to tell you concerning your diagnosis and prognosis.   T_____ F_____

8. Your doctor is obligated to tell you all the risks involved in any course of treatment he proposes.   T_____ F_____

9. A hospital can keep you on a life-support system regardless of your wishes or those of your family.   T_____ F_____

10. You have the right to refuse to be discharged even if your doctor says it is safe for you to go home.   T_____ F_____

11. You have the right to review your medical record without charge.   T_____ F_____

12. You may be open to a lawsuit by your doctor if you report her improper care to the hospital administration.   T_____ F_____

ANSWERS:

1- T
2- F
3- F
4- T
5- F
6- F
7- F
8- T
9- F
10- T
11- T
12- F

*The following
is an example
of one state's
patient's bill of rights*

New York State Patient's Bill of Rights

As a patient in a hospital, YOU HAVE THE RIGHT to:

1. understand and use these rights. If for any reason you do not understand or you need help, the hospital must provide assistance, including an interpreter.

2. receive treatment without discrimination as to race, color, religion, sex, national origin, disability, sexual orientation, or source of payment.

3. receive considerate and respectful care in a clean and safe environment free of unnecessary restraints.

4. receive emergency care if you need it.

5. be informed of the name and position of the doctor who will be in charge of your care in the hospital.

6. know the names, positions, and functions of any hospital staff involved in your care and refuse their treatment, examination or observation.

7. a no-smoking room.

8. receive complete information about your diagnosis, treatment and prognosis.

9. receive all the information that you need to give informed consent for any proposed procedure or treatment. This information shall include the possible risks and benefits of the procedure or treatment.

10. receive all information you need to give informed consent for an order not to resuscitate. You also have the right to designate an individual to give this consent for you if you are too ill to do so. If you would like additional information, please ask for a copy of the pamphlet, "Do Not Resuscitate Orders — A Guide for Patients and Families."

11. refuse treatment and be told what effect this may have on your health.

12. refuse to take part in research. In deciding whether or not to participate, you have the right to a full explanation.

13. privacy while in the hospital and confidentiality of all information and records regarding your care.

14. participate in all decisions about your treatment and discharge from the hospital. The hospital must provide you with a written discharge plan and written description of how you can appeal your discharge.

15. review your medical record without charge and obtain a copy of your medical record for which the hospital can charge a reasonable fee. You cannot be denied a copy solely because you cannot afford to pay.

16. receive an itemized bill and explanation of all charges.

17. complain without fear of reprisals about the care and services you are receiving and to have the hospital respond to you and, if you request it, a written response. If you are not satisfied with the hospital's response, you can complain to the New York State Health Department. The hospital must provide you with the Health Department telephone number.

SECTION ONE

YOUR RIGHTS AS A PATIENT IN A MEDICAL EMERGENCY

You are lying in a hospital emergency room, having just suffered a serious accident, stroke, heart attack or some other medical trauma. For the moment, you are so frightened and worried that you are only too willing to turn over all decisions regarding your medical care to unknown doctors.

This is the only time you need to unconditionally accept a doctor's recommendation.

As soon as your condition becomes stabilized, you should begin exercising YOUR RIGHTS AS A PATIENT. Keep in mind that you must never consent to any treatment, test or medication unless you fully understand both the risks and benefits involved.

Your Right to Question
or Refuse Diagnostic Tests

YOU HAVE THE RIGHT to understand what diagnostic tests will be performed and why these tests were prescribed prior to giving your "informed consent." The hospital must get your written permission before performing any invasive tests (such as injecting a dye into your system). Therefore, prior to signing such a release, it is essential that you discuss with your doctor all ramifications of the test.

When discussing diagnostic tests, remember to be prepared with a list of questions and take notes. Basic questions should include the following:

- What is the purpose of the test?
- What risks are involved in taking (or delaying) the test?
- Are there any potential side effects?
- Is there a less dangerous test that would provide the same information?
- When will you discuss the results with me?

If there is any doubt about either the necessity or the safety of a test, you should insist on obtaining a second opinion from another doctor of your choice unless a delay would result in a life-threatening situation.

Your Right to a Second Opinion

YOU HAVE THE RIGHT and responsibility to seek a second opinion if there is any doubt concerning testing, diagnosis or treatment. The concept of obtaining second (and even third) opinions is so generally accepted these days that many insurance companies actually require them before surgery. Even though you use an outside consultant, you can still continue to be under the care of your original physician.

When beginning the search for a second opinion, it is important to find a doctor whose particular strengths within a specialty match your medical problem. Remember, within every specialty there are many subspecialties. For example, ophthalmologists can be experts in areas as varied as cataracts, glaucoma, or plastic surgery.

Brian's Story

Baby Brian was diagnosed by a neurosurgeon as having an inoperable brain tumor, which would cause his death within a few months. His parents had assumed that, because the doctor was a neurosurgeon, he was qualified to diagnose and treat their son. Nevertheless, they couldn't accept this death sentence without getting at least one more opinion. After making many inquiries, the parents located a *pediatric* neurosurgeon. This doctor believed the tumor could be removed. As a result, that "hopeless" infant is now a healthy, active youngster.

When seeking a consultant for a second opinion, there are several ways to locate an appropriate doctor.

- Your family doctor can refer you to other physicians. You must be sure to ask whether this recommendation is based on first-hand knowledge or only on hearsay.
- University teaching hospitals are excellent sources for consultants, because doctors there often face greater medical challenges and tougher problems than in community hospitals.
- Self-help organizations (groups serving people with strokes, cancer, head injuries, etc.) have names of doctors on file that their members have recommended.
- Medical societies can provide names of specialists who are board certified. However, this gives you no information about these individuals or how they are ranked by their peers.

YOU HAVE THE RIGHT to check the qualifications of any doctor you are considering as a consultant, by asking the following questions:
- Is he board certified?
- What is her record and experience in treating
  your particular medical problem?
- How long has the doctor practiced?
- How many years has he practiced in the
  same location? (You might wonder about a
  doctor who has moved from state to state.)

Your Right to Reject a "Hopeless" Verdict

YOU HAVE THE RIGHT to reject a verdict that your situation is hopeless until all other options have been explored.

Katharine's Story

Katharine H., a woman in her late 50's, had been troubled for several weeks by tingling and numbness in her arms and hands. Finally, after gardening all day, she experienced an excruciating, stabbing pain in the back of her neck. Thinking that she had a badly pinched nerve, she asked a friend to drive her to a nearby hospital. By the time she arrived, her legs had begun to tremble uncontrollably and she was admitted to the emergency room for observation.

The next morning, Katharine had become totally paralyzed from the neck down and needed a respirator in order to breathe. The hospital's neurologists determined that she had a blood clot on her spinal cord, between the third and fourth cervical vertebrae, a very rare occurrence that is almost always fatal.

Katharine's adult children were told by the senior neurologist that there was little chance their mother could live, and, if she were "unfortunate enough to survive," she would be completely paralyzed, unable even to speak. The doctor urged her children to authorize the removal of her respirator.

Her family was unwilling to give up so quickly and instead located a neurologist with an outstanding reputation who agreed to give a second opinion. After examining the woman, the consultant stated that he believed she had a 50-50 chance of surviving. However, because there was also a strong possibility that she would remain permanently paralyzed from the neck down, he advised that the patient be allowed to make up her own mind about whether she wanted to stay on the respirator. She decided not to give up, no matter what the eventual outcome might be.

Within six weeks, she could breathe unaided and, after nine months of intensive physical and occupational therapy, she regained almost full use of her right side and partial control of her left side. Although she continues to require the assistance of a personal care aide and visiting nurse, she now leads an active and fulfilling life. In fact, she is one of the authors of this book, Katharine Halkin.

Your Right to Be
Fully Informed by Doctors

YOU HAVE THE RIGHT to receive complete information from your doctor about your diagnosis, treatment, and prognosis. When requesting information, remember that doctors, like all people, vary in personality; some are more pleasant and approachable than others. Although obtaining the information you need is often a frustrating process, you can't afford to be hostile.   You are under stress, but the doctor probably is, too, because he has the responsibility of caring for many seriously ill patients.

Staying calm gets the best results.

Be organized.

Your doctor's time is very limited; therefore, it's important to be clear and focused when speaking to him. Since visiting hours often do not coincide with the times that doctors make their rounds, families can communicate with doctors either by phone, in a pre-arranged meeting or by leaving a written note with ICU nurses. When you are talking with a doctor, prepare all your questions in advance and keep a record of all responses. Additional suggestions for effectively communicating with doctors can be found in Section Two of this book.

Your Right to Transfer to Another Hospital

Selecting a Hospital

YOU HAVE THE RIGHT to transfer to a different hospital if you feel this is advisable. There are a number of situations that could lead to this decision, including the following:

- The present hospital lacks the facilities for testing and/or treatment that you need.
- You wish to continue with a consulting physician and he is not affiliated with your hospital.
- Another hospital in the area specializes in treating your medical problem.
- Another hospital is equally suitable but is more conveniently located for family members and others you will be depending on.

If you wish to transfer to another hospital, there are several good ways to locate and select a suitable facility.

- Look for a university teaching hospital or one that is connected with a medical school. This is generally the best choice.
- Seek the advice of your doctor and other specialists.
- Contact local support groups. (These groups are not only places where you can receive emotional support but also invaluable resources for a wide variety of up-to-date information.)
- At the very least, a hospital should be accredited by the Joint Commission on Hospital Accreditation.
- Call your county medical society.

YOU HAVE THE RIGHT to question the frequency and success rate in treating your particular medical problems for all hospitals you are considering.

Hospitals now keep performance statistics, which should be available to you just for the asking. But, if you are unable to get this information, ask your doctor for help. You can also contact the regional office of the U.S. Department of Health and Human Services.

Making the Transfer

When you transfer to another hospital, the admitting doctor and doctors from your present hospital will take care of medical details. However, transportation details are usually handled by the social work staff from the first hospital. If you are transferring against the hospital's recommendation or if you disagree with the selected mode of transportation, you may be expected to contact the transportation carrier and handle all related matters. If this happens, be sure to ask the new hospital which form of transportation is best for your needs.

Unless other arrangements are made, the ambulance company may request payment at the time of transfer. If funds are not available, you should see if the hospital social worker can arrange some alternate method of payment.

Finally, some member of the family will probably have to be at the new hospital to admit the patient. (Check on this in advance.)

Barbara's Story

Barbara encountered just about every problem that a patient could face when planning to transfer to another hospital. She had fallen from her second floor porch when the wooden railing she was leaning against gave way and had sustained multiple fractures to her head, back, ribs, arms and face. After emergency medical care and testing had been completed at a small local hospital, the hospital indicated that surgery was necessary and recommended transfer to another community hospital that had a thoracic surgeon on staff. Her sons disagreed with this choice, preferring that she go to a major metropolitan teaching hospital, where they believed she would receive more expert treatment. When they discussed these feelings with their mother, she agreed and asked them to handle the details.

Because the family had intervened and made their own choice, the first hospital ceased to be involved with the transfer except to order an ambulance for the twenty-five-mile trip into the city.

Her sons had to intervene once again when the city hospital advised them that traveling in an ambulance would be unsafe, given the extent of their mother's injuries. The second hospital recommended that she be transferred by their helicopter.

More problems arose when her insurance company initially refused to cover the cost of a helicopter, until her two sons prevailed upon the admitting doctor to write a strong letter justifying the need. On the day of the transfer, one son had to stay at the community hospital until his mother left, to make certain there were no problems or last minute papers to be signed, while his brother waited at the new hospital to help with the admitting process. It was this initial experience in a recovery process, which included months of hospitalization, that led Barbara Hardt, one of the authors of this book, to the realization that understanding one's rights as a patient directly affects the quality of one's care.

Your Right to Adequate Nursing in ICU

YOU HAVE THE RIGHT to adequate nursing care when you are a patient in an intensive care unit (ICU) or a coronary care unit (CCU). Patients are placed within sight of medical staff at all times and can usually count on getting care whenever it is medically necessary. However, in the rare instances when this level of care is not adequate to meet the needs of patients with special problems, families may have to intervene.

James' Story

James R. suffered such a severe stroke that he was soon unable to breathe. He was given a tracheotomy and put on a respirator. Because of the tracheotomy, James formed large amounts of mucous that had to be extracted every fifteen to twenty minutes by suctioning in order to prevent him from choking. Unfortunately, three other critical cases were admitted to the unit within the next twelve hours, and the nurses were not always able to suction James as frequently as was required.

Mrs. R. asked the doctor to obtain permission for her to stay at her husband's bedside continuously in order to assist him, despite the hospital's policy of only allowing visitors into ICU four times a day for twenty minutes. Although this was an unusual request, the hospital approved it because of the unique circumstances.

Your Right to Receive Assistance in Communicating

YOU HAVE THE RIGHT to receive assistance in communicating if you are hearing impaired, unable to speak, or do not speak English. When patients are admitted to a hospital emergency room in a life threatening situation, there is usually no time to obtain the services of translators for non-English-speaking people or sign language interpreters for those who are deaf. Likewise, it is difficult to find ways to immediately help persons who are unable to speak.

However, once these patients are transferred from the emergency room to an intensive care unit, a method of communication must be established.

Helping a patient who cannot speak to express himself calls for a bit of creativity. Even patients who are paralyzed can often blink their eyes or nod their heads to answer "yes" or "no" questions. Large hospitals usually have speech departments where staff or families can obtain communication devices. Where this service is not available, the families of patients with speech and language impairments may have to devise their own methods.

Hospitals are required to provide the services of a sign language interpreter for hearing impaired patients. (Written communication can only be used as a temporary measure.) Hospitals are also obliged to provide translators for non-English-speaking persons. However, if no one is immediately available to perform this function, family members or friends should be allowed to be present as often as their services are needed. For patients who speak a little-known language, hospital staff should ask bilingual visitors to write out key medical phrases phonetically in the person's language and post this "dictionary" above the bed. Assistance can also be sought from public or private agencies that serve hard-of-hearing and foreign-born people.

Keep in mind that nonprofessional translators may not be able to relate sensitive information in a manner that is both correct and nonthreatening.

Miguel's Story

Miguel G., an elderly man who lived alone, fell on the ice when returning home one evening. A bystander called 911, and Miguel was taken to the emergency room of a nearby hospital. When he arrived at the emergency room, he was in a great deal of pain and was very frightened because he could not walk. He could speak no English and none of the doctors and nurses on duty that night spoke Spanish.

The orthopedic surgeon who was called in to examine Miguel determined that his right hip was broken and that surgery would be required to repair the damage. In order to perform this operation, he needed Miguel's written permission. After a number of futile attempts to explain the situation, the doctor finally asked a nurse to find someone who was bilingual to serve as a translator. The nearest available person was a hospital orderly. When the doctor asked him to tell Miguel that he needed surgery, the orderly let his own fear of surgery color his translation. As a result,

Miguel became even more agitated and nothing further could be done about getting permission for the operation until the hospital's bilingual social worker came to work the following morning.

Had the emergency room staff and the orthopedist been able to locate a translator with a professional background, Miguel would have been spared many hours of anguish.

Involving Hospital Social Workers

Most hospitals have social work departments that can be extremely helpful to patients and their families during a medical emergency. The social work staff can assist you in the following ways:

- Provide counseling to patients and family members who express difficulty in coping with hospitalization.

- Provide information on how to contact other hospital departments and personnel, such as patient advocates and chaplains.

- Provide information about relevant support groups.

- Make transportation arrangements (if you are transferring with hospital approval), or provide names of ambulance companies.

- Help patients to apply for Medicaid.

- Provide information regarding Workers' Compensation, Social Security Disability Insurance, and other benefits.

- Develop discharge plans for patients to enable them to leave the hospital with all necessary services arranged for.

Preparing for Private Duty Care

Before you leave ICU, you must make arrangements for the care you will need once you are transferred to a regular floor. If you are very weak and unable to get out of bed, feed yourself or wash yourself, be aware that the floor nurses may not be available to assist you as often as you would like. Many hospitals are understaffed and are unable to give the amount of personalized care that seriously ill patients require. If this is the case, your doctor may be able to help by requesting that you be placed close to the nurses' station.

You should also consider arranging to have someone at your bedside for as long as you need extra care. Some hospitals even provide cots so that family members can stay overnight with patients. If this is not possible, either because of hospital regulations or because no one is available, you can hire a registered nurse (RN), licensed practical nurse (LPN), or nurse's aide.

Having additional care during this time should not be looked on as an unnecessary luxury. If there is a question about whether your insurance company will reimburse this expense, a doctor's letter, stating that the hospital staff cannot adequately attend to your needs, can often resolve the issue.

The hospital's nursing office will discuss with your family the procedures for arranging for private duty care. Some hospitals will make these arrangements, but others expect the families to assume this responsibility. Many hospitals have a directory of recommended nurses; if yours does not, it is important to contact a reliable health care agency. Staff nurses can often give you names of good agencies or you can ask the hospital social worker. Nursing agencies generally have pre-set shifts for their employees, but if a different schedule is required, they may make the necessary accommodations.

Summary

- Unless you are in a life or death situation with no time to question a doctor's treatment, you should always take the time to ensure that you are not being deprived of your PATIENT'S RIGHTS.
- YOU HAVE THE RIGHT to understand the purpose of all tests and THE RIGHT to refuse to take a test if you doubt the necessity or fear the risks.
- YOU HAVE THE RIGHT to a second opinion and you should only seek doctors experienced in treating your particular medical problem.
- YOU HAVE THE RIGHT to reject a "hopeless" diagnosis unless all avenues have been explored.
- Avoid hostile situations when talking to doctors, no matter how frustrated you feel, and remain clear and focused in order to maximize your time with them.
- YOU HAVE THE RIGHT to receive complete information from your doctor, so be prepared with a list of questions and write down all answers.

- YOU HAVE THE RIGHT to transfer to another hospital, and you should if it's better equipped to help you.
- YOU HAVE THE RIGHT to adequate care in ICU.
- YOU HAVE THE RIGHT to an interpreter if you are hearing impaired or do not speak English.
- Hospital social workers can be helpful in many ways.
- Before leaving ICU, arrangements for private nursing care should be considered.

SECTION TWO

YOUR RIGHTS AS A PATIENT DURING NONEMERGENCY HOSPITALIZATION

You come to a hospital to get well. Yet, even if you are in an excellent hospital and have a highly respected doctor, things can still go wrong.

You must be actively involved in the management of your own case, because your life can depend on it.

As a hospital patient, YOU HAVE THE RIGHT to question and understand all aspects of your treatment before you give your approval. This is what is meant by "informed consent." Unfortunately, too many patients sign consent forms without understanding the risks, benefits or possible alternative procedures available.

Your Right to Be Fully Informed by Your Doctor

YOU HAVE THE RIGHT to be fully informed by your doctor about your condition, treatment and prognosis. In order to ensure this right, you must be organized and clear about the information you require.

- Write down everything you wish to discuss.
- Give your doctor a list of any changes you are requesting (i.e., being allowed out of bed, different medications or diet), so he won't forget to enter them on your chart.
- Be sure to include your name on any written communications.

If you have designated a family member to speak to your doctor on your behalf this person should tape a note for the doctor in a place where it will easily be seen, asking him to call and listing times when the family member will be available. The note should specify exactly what they want to discuss.

Whenever possible, record all in-person and telephone conversations, because we tend to forget details, especially when under stress. The ideal situation is to have another person present when talking to your doctor so there is someone to take notes on the doctor's responses to your questions. If there is no one to help out, you could use a tape recorder, with permission, so you won't have to worry about taking notes. The doctor should understand and appreciate this technique, because it will save time and eliminate misunderstandings.

Paul's Story

Paul T. was struck down by a young cyclist while taking his daily walk in the park. Upon being rushed to the hospital, he was given a complete series of x-rays and a CT (CAT) scan. These tests indicated that he had broken his left leg and hip and would probably require surgery. However, Paul was unwilling to accept the seriousness of his condition and was frightened about undergoing what he felt was a dangerous operation.

Because of his resistance, Paul's wife asked the hospital's orthopedic surgeon if he would meet with them to discuss the purpose and ramifications of the operation. The doctor interpreted the x-rays for the couple and explained how surgery would correct Paul's problem and what the recuperative process would entail. Once Paul fully understood his medical condition, he consented to surgery with no further qualms.

Your Right to Monitor Your Medications

YOU HAVE THE RIGHT to know the names and purpose of all medications you are taking.

YOU HAVE THE RIGHT to refuse any medication you feel is harmful.

Jane's Story

After a serious accident, Jane R. was admitted to the hospital. Upon admission, she listed the medications she was taking daily, including one to control her high blood pressure. However, as a result of the accident, her blood pressure actually became dangerously low. When Jane asked the nurse to tell her the name and purpose of all medications being given to her, she discovered that she was still getting the medication to control high blood pressure! She immediately refused to take this medicine and asked to speak to the doctor, who then discontinued the drug.

Jane did not make the mistake of passively accepting, without question, her medications. She took responsibility for assuming an active role in her own treatment and probably saved her life as a result.

Remember, you have the right to refuse any medication that you feel is harmful.

A Word of Caution

Once each day, most hospital pharmacies dispense to the nursing stations all medications that patients take during a twenty-four-hour period. However, if the pharmacy is out of a particular medication, you may miss one or more doses until a new supply arrives. Your nurse is supposed to take note of this fact, but the possibility exists that, when the medicine finally comes, she may forget to give you the makeup dose. Therefore, it's up to you to remind her. However, you need to understand that certain medications cannot be given at a later time, for a variety of reasons, so don't get upset if your nurse explains that a makeup dose is not recommended. If requested, some hospitals will give patients printouts of the relevant facts about medications.

Pain Medication

Pain medication can be a major cause of contro-
versy between doctors and patients and, if possible, this subject should be discussed prior to hospitalization. Any patient who knows he cannot tol-
erate certain types of pain medication should
immediately convey this information to the attending physician. One new self-medicating system,
known as patient-controlled analgesia or PCA,
permits the patient to administer her own medication up to previously programmed limits. Additional suggestions on how to take charge of your
own doses of pain medication are discussed on
pages 48 and 49.

Your Right to Monitor Tests and Procedures

As emphasized in Section One, it is essential to question the purpose and results of diagnostic tests such as CT (CAT) scans, MRIs, spinal taps, blood tests, etc. However, don't ignore the fact that each time someone takes your blood pressure, pulse, temperature, or other routine index of your health, YOU HAVE THE RIGHT to know these results as well and should ask for them each time.

Sally's Story

When Sally G. had a heart attack, she informed the doctor that she took insulin injections to control her diabetes and the doctor, therefore, prescribed a continuation of this treatment. However, after two weeks her blood-sugar level began to drop dramatically because her restricted hospital diet contained far less sugar and other carbohydrates than she normally ate at home. Even though a nurse tested Sally's blood sugar level every day, and recorded the fact that it had dropped substantially, other nurses continued to give Sally her regular insulin dosage, which was now too high.

As a result, Sally went into insulin shock one night. In spite of this, the next morning a nurse came to administer the same dosage of insulin to Sally. At that point, it became obvious to her that there was a serious reporting problem between the various nursing shifts and that she could not assume that she was automatically receiving the proper insulin dosage. Therefore, Sally informed the nurses that she wanted to know the results of her daily blood-sugar test before consenting to an injection.

Your Right to Monitor Your Diet

The hospital dietitian is supposed to follow your doctor's orders regarding the type of food you receive, according to your particular dietetic restrictions, if any. YOU HAVE THE RIGHT to know what diet your doctor prescribed and to question it if you feel it is not appropriate. Once you have mutually agreed on a diet, make certain that the menus you receive each day conform to your doctor's orders.

If you've ever been in a hospital, you know that dietary mistakes can occasionally occur. Nurses generally don't see your trays, and the aides or orderlies who deliver them have no information about your diet. Always check the name and room number on your tray to be sure it belongs to you.

Annette's Story

Annette G. was a twenty-three-year-old woman with Down Syndrome. When she was admitted to the hospital for corrective orthopedic surgery, her mother, Helen, was asked if Annette was allergic to any medications or foods. Helen replied that Annette had very serious reactions to cooked tomatoes and shellfish. This fact was relayed to the hospital's dietitian.

However, that evening a nurses' aide accidentally gave Annette a shrimp Creole dinner that another patient had ordered. Not understanding the danger, Annette began to eat this food. Fortunately, her nurse came in and corrected the mistake. As soon as Helen learned of the incident, she placed a note listing her daughter's food allergies above Annette's bed.

Your Right to Adequate Nursing Care

Although it's understood that you will receive less nursing care on a regular floor than patients receive in ICU or in the recovery room after surgery, most people are not prepared for how little nursing care they may actually receive if a hospital is understaffed.

Nevertheless YOU HAVE THE RIGHT to adequate nursing care.

If your doctor prescribes a level of nursing care that the regular nursing staff cannot provide, you will have to find some way to resolve this problem. The hospital's patient advocate or social worker can often be of help.

Ed's Story

A week after an automobile accident that caused multiple fractures of his legs, arms, and ribs, Ed J. was transferred from the intensive care unit to a regular hospital bed. A few days later, he began to have difficulty breathing. An x-ray disclosed that his lungs were filled with fluid and, even after being drained, the fluid continued to accumulate.

The hospital's pulmonary specialist offered two options: corrective surgery or a very aggressive pulmonary exercise regime, to be done at thirty minute intervals. Ed was willing to do anything to avoid surgery, but it was apparent after the first day that the floor nurses were not always available to assist him every thirty minutes. Ed informed the hospital's pulmonary specialist that he was not receiving the level of care that had been prescribed.

In order to avoid surgery, he asked the doctor to either get approval from his insurance company to have a private nurse or to return him to ICU, where more nursing care would be available. Because of the seriousness of Ed's condition, his insurance company approved private nursing care. They realized that either surgery or returning to the ICU would have been much more costly.

The type of nursing you will require depends on your specific medical problem.

Private Duty Nurses

Having a private duty nurse is the optimum choice for seriously ill patients. Section One describes the necessary steps for obtaining this care, including the role your doctor needs to play in order to obtain approval from your insurance company.

Having a good relationship with your private nurse is essential, but, for a variety of reasons, this does not always happen. If you're not satisfied with a nurse's performance, you should talk it over immediately. If this doesn't work, chalk it up to bad chemistry and request a replacement for the next day.

It is not always necessary to use a registered nurse (RN) for private duty care. Some hospitals allow patients to hire licensed practical nurses (LPNs) or even nurses aides for this purpose.

"Civilian" Nurses

If there is absolutely no way you can afford private nursing care, someone close to you may be
willing to assist. Many hospitals actually encour-
age this practice and will provide cots for
caregivers, and other necessary services.

Floor Nurses

Whether you have a private duty nurse or a "civilian" nurse, you will also have to interact with hospital nurses, if only for dispensing medication. And, eventually, once you no longer require special nursing care, you will be totally dependent on floor nurses. Therefore, it is essential that you know how to develop a good relationship with the hospital nurses assigned to you.

Don't be just another lump lying in a bed!

Nurses will only get to know you as an individual when you start relating to them in a personal way. Make a point of learning their names. Try to be pleasant, no matter how miserable you may be feeling. Be sure to thank your nurses (and all hospital staff) each time they do something that makes you comfortable. When you are strong enough, involve them in conversations that are not just related to your illness. Getting to know your nurses has an added advantage. Most nurses are invaluable sources of medical information as well as excellent liaisons between you and hospital doctors.

You will earn the undying gratitude of the floor nurses if you do not waste their time. Many hospitals are seriously understaffed, so maximizing the limited time a nurse can give you is essential. Make a list (actual or mental) of all the things you require, so the nurse can do everything during just one visit to your room.

A Patient's Nightmare

Nurse Ratchit is assigned to your room! She is the type of person who thrives on being in control of helpless patients. Her one saving grace is that she only works eight hours a day, but if she is really making your life miserable and therefore interfering with your healing, there are steps you can take.

- Try to establish a personal relationship. Complimenting her indirectly by asking her opinion on a medical subject may soften her up.
- If you feel capable of dealing with the problem directly, tell her how her attitude is affecting you and ask her to let up.
- If you can't resolve the situation by yourself, you should talk to the nursing supervisor about moving to a different room and/or having a different nurse assigned to you.

Nurses and Pain Medication

Although doctors prescribe pain medication and nurses dispense it, most people don't realize that, along with the type of medication prescribed, there are options the patient can exercise regarding dosage and intervals.

YOU HAVE THE RIGHT to ask the following questions:

- What kind of pain medication is prescribed for me?
- What is the range of dosage I'm allowed ?
- What is the least amount of time allowed between doses?
- Are there any side effects I should be aware of?

It is only after you have taken several doses of pain medication that you can begin to evaluate its effectiveness in terms of how much you need and how often. Once you learn how your body responds to the medication prescribed for you, you can request it according to your needs, within the limits of the doctor's prescription. (If necessary, you can ask your doctor to make adjustments, based on your response to the original prescription.)

Unfortunately, some nurses have attitudes and biases regarding pain medication, and will try to control dispensing your medication according to what *they* feel is appropriate.

YOU MUST ASSERT YOUR RIGHT to receive your medication as you have determined you need it.

Bob's Story

Bob H. was receiving heavy doses of morphine every three to four hours to manage his pain. Although the morphine made the pain bearable, after the first day Bob started to hallucinate and became violent. He was understandably disturbed by this reaction and asked the nurse if she thought the dosage was too strong. The nurse informed him that the doctor had prescribed the morphine within a range of incremental doses of 1 to 5 and that he was receiving the maximum amount. Bob then requested that the next dose be lowered to 2. When this lower dosage was administered, Bob was relieved to find that his pain could be managed without the extreme side effects he had previously experienced with the more potent dose.

Helping Patients Who Cannot Speak, Are Hearing Impaired or Do Not Speak English, and Their Right to an Interpreter

Nonverbal Patients

There are a number of ways to help patients who are unable to speak to communicate. If the hospital has a speech department, they may have number and letter charts, as well as pictures of basic patient needs, which staff and family members can use with the patient. (The hospital social worker can contact the speech department for you.) If not, these tools are easy to make or buy. Toy stores sell alphabet and number boards, and the family can draw activity pictures, using stick figures, or can cut pictures from magazines and mount them on cardboard. When a patient is unable to point to a letter or picture, others do the pointing and the patient can signify what is correct by whatever means possible: an eye blink, nod of the head, or any noise she can make.

It is imperative that nonverbal patients have ways to signal when they need help. Resolving this problem as quickly as possible will do much to lessen a patient's (and family's) fears and frustrations.

Diane's Story

Diane S. sustained an injury to her spinal cord in a diving accident and became paralyzed from the neck down. After she was transferred out of the intensive care unit to a regular floor, her parents hired a private duty nurse to stay with her when they could not be at her bedside.

After a few weeks, when there was no longer a need for this extra care, the special nurse was discharged. However, before this service was discontinued, Mr. and Mrs. S. realized that Diane would have no way of signalling the floor nurse when she needed help. Their daughter was unable to speak and couldn't move her fingers to press a call bell.

Mrs. S. asked the hospital social worker to assist them. The social worker contacted one of the hospital's engineers, who designed a large call button Diane could activate with her head. This simple but essential device made it possible for Diane to be left alone without fear that she could not summon help when it was needed.

Hearing Impaired Patients

Hospitals must provide the services of a sign-language interpreter for patients who have hearing impairments. In an emergency, the hospital may have to communicate information in writing, but this method cannot be used as a permanent solution.

Non-English-Speaking Patients

Non-English-speaking patients have an even greater problem because they can neither understand nor be understood. Although YOU HAVE THE RIGHT to a bilingual interpreter, hospitals often do not employ professional translators and thus may have to use anyone on staff who is available. However, if these individuals are not capable of conveying sensitive or complex information, the patient could be subjected to unnecessary stress.

Other options that hospitals can take include the following:

- Bilingual family members and friends can be requested to post a schedule over the patient's bed listing the times when they will be available, either in person or by phone, for consultation and translation.
- The hospital can ask family members or friends to phonetically write out words for all medical phrases that are needed for the care of a patient with a particular medical problem.
- The hospital could subscribe to a commercial service that connects non-English-speaking patients to translators by phone.

Obtaining Other Professional Services

Hospitals usually have a variety of professionals who can be of assistance to you and your family. In addition to social workers (whose roles are explained in Section One of this book), you can also request help from psychologists, psychiatrists, rehabilitation therapists, dietitians, and chaplains. If you are in doubt about how to contact any of these individuals, your social worker or floor nurse can help you. Sometimes, patients have concerns that can't be solved by these professionals. However, most hospitals provide a grievance or complaint mechanism and some hospitals even employ patient representatives who can find the most appropriate solution to the problems of patients.

YOU HAVE THE RIGHT to know the names, positions and functions of any hospital staff involved in your care. YOU ALSO HAVE THE RIGHT to refuse their treatment, examination or observation.

Alice's Story

Alice W. was recuperating from a mild stroke. After four weeks of hospitalization, she was well enough to be transferred to the hospital's rehabilitation section. As a matter of course in this hospital, all patients undergoing rehabilitation are assigned to a psychologist who administers a series of cognitive tests and provides counseling. Alice was very uncomfortable with the young psychologist assigned to her and thus lacked confidence in this individual. She requested a more mature psychologist who, she believed, could better understand her problems. Although Alice may have misjudged the first psychologist, she nevertheless had the right to request someone different.

Your Right to Considerate and Respectful Treatment

YOU HAVE THE RIGHT to receive considerate and respectful care in a clean and safe environment.

Just because you are an invalid doesn't mean that people should treat you as if you are in-VALID.

Bedside Manners

Unfortunately, there are some doctors who forget that they need to be sensitive to patients' feelings. Don't be afraid to tell doctors and other medical personnel that you don't like the way they are treating you. YOU HAVE A RIGHT to know the names and functions of all people who care for you and you can report those individuals who do not treat you with consideration.

If you are in a teaching hospital, in all probability you will eventually find one or more classes of medical students gathered around your bedside while a professor discusses your case so objectively you may begin to feel like a nonperson. YOU HAVE THE RIGHT to refuse their examinations and you should let them know immediately if their probing hurts you or if their comments upset you. Should this happen, contact your doctor or the chief resident and ask him to see that you are not disturbed in this way again.

Karen's Story

Karen W. had just been transferred from ICU to a regular hospital bed. When the nurse was getting her settled, the resident on duty walked in. Stethoscope in hand, he turned to the nurse and asked, "Can she sit up?"

"Yes," snapped Karen, "and I can hear and speak, too!"

Roommate Etiquette

You should ask the floor nurse or your doctor to place you in a different room if you have a roommate who:

- has more noisy visitors than hospital regulations permit;
- talks incessantly when you are trying to sleep;
- in any other way creates an environment that is not conducive to your healing.

The Discharge Process and Your Right to Appeal

There are two parts to the discharge process: the discharge notice and the discharge plan.

The Discharge Notice

Determining when you are ready to leave the hospital is far more complicated than just evaluating your medical condition. Although your health needs are the primary consideration, the hospital must also abide by the dictates outlined in your DRG category. DRG (Diagnostic Related Groups) is a federally mandated system for Medicare reimbursement. It categorizes treatment according to particular medical conditions, such as cardiac problems or pulmonary problems. The maximum amount of time and cost allowed to treat each medical problem is predetermined, based on the average expense of similar cases, and can only be increased if the hospital can demonstrate serious extenuating circumstances. Insurance companies often tie their own coverage to these DRG time frames — in some states they are required to — and therefore will only reimburse hospitals for the number of days authorized by a DRG.

Your attending physician may tell you when you are to be discharged, but in any event you will receive a written discharge notice giving the date of your discharge. If you think that you are not ready to leave the hospital, this notice contains specific instructions on how to exercise YOUR RIGHT TO APPEAL.

If your hospital costs are covered by Medicare, the name of your patient advocate will be included as part of your discharge notice. This person should be contacted if you have any concerns about your discharge.

So long as you follow these instructions, you will not have to pay for additional days in the hospital (up to three) while your appeal is under review.

Sam's Story

When seventy-four year-old Sam R. was discharged from the hospital only three days after his hernia operation, he and his wife accepted his discharge notice without question. Sam was so weak he could hardly speak or step from the wheelchair into his car. After only twelve hours at home, Sam collapsed in the bathroom, struck his head on the sink, and had to be rushed back to the hospital. He never regained consciousness, and died two days later.

The tragic irony of this case is that the discharge notice Sam received included very specific instructions stating that HE HAD THE RIGHT to appeal the proposed date of discharge if he disagreed with it. But Sam was so anxious and confused that he didn't read the notice before he signed it. If he had requested an appeal, he would have been allowed to remain in the hospital for up to three days while his case was being reviewed. Sam's medical insurance would have been required to cover his stay, thus allowing him more time to recuperate.

The Discharge Plan

YOU HAVE THE RIGHT to receive a written discharge plan before leaving the hospital. This must include a description of arrangements made for your future health care once you leave the hospital.

The services that patients may require include part-time skilled nursing care, home health aides, a wide range of equipment, therapy services, home modifications, or discharge to a nursing home.

You should not agree to being discharged until the services outlined in your written discharge plan are secured or are determined by you and the hospital to be reasonably available.

If you are dissatisfied, YOU HAVE THE RIGHT to appeal your discharge plan. If you follow the appeal process correctly, you are allowed up to three additional days in the hospital, at no cost to you, while your appeal is under review.

Theresa's Story

Theresa B. was recovering from a serious illness and could not yet be cared for at home. Her doctor therefore prescribed placement in a nursing home. The hospital's discharge planner made arrangements at a facility that Theresa and her family felt was not as suitable as other nursing homes in the area. However, the homes that Theresa wanted to go to had no beds immediately available and it appeared that she had no choice but to go along with the discharge plan. Nevertheless, they exercised THEIR RIGHT TO APPEAL the discharge plan, and provided the review agent with documentation that proved their contention that the home selected by the discharge planner was inappropriate for Theresa. She was therefore allowed to stay in the hospital until a bed became available at one of the other facilities.

Getting the Most from Your Medical Insurance Policy

When you first entered the hospital, the admitting office checked to see that you had coverage for hospitalization. However, you also need to determine exactly what other services are covered by your policy. The first source of information is the policy itself, but the wording is often unclear. For clarification, contact the company directly, but also talk to your insurance agent, your employer's personnel director, or your union representative, for their interpretations. Take careful notes, including the names and titles of the persons to whom you speak. If possible, be sure to have all statements put in writing. If not, send a registered letter to your contact, summarizing the key points that were made.

These safeguards are essential in order to avoid confusion or a denial of coverage at a later date.

If you are denied a service you really need, don't accept "no" for an answer unless you've tried every possible approach. Your doctor can often make things right, but even if she cannot, there are additional things you can do. It always helps to talk to someone who has the power to make decisions.

Michelle's Story

Michelle B. needed plastic surgery on her eye in order to restore muscles damaged by an accident. Her insurance company refused to pay for this operation, explaining that her policy did not cover eye surgery. Michelle phoned the company and gained the sympathy of a receptionist, who referred her to a supervisor who had the authority to make exceptions. Upon learning the reason for the surgery, the supervisor gave her approval.

Regardless of how limited your health insurance policy may appear, there is always room for negotiation, especially if you can demonstrate that what you need, even if it is not covered by your plan, will actually save the insurance company money.

Never assume that any insurance policy is written in stone.

Insurance companies make exceptions every day for a variety of reasons. YOU HAVE A RIGHT to try to negotiate for any service you legitimately need.

Arlene's Story

During her fifteen years of marriage, Arlene J.'s physical condition had progressively deteriorated as a result of a series of operations to remove tumors from her spine. She had changed from an active, vigorous person to one who could barely walk a few steps. Because of her condition, she had given up all hope of having children. So, when she learned she was pregnant, Arlene and her husband were ecstatic, but they were also very worried because of her physical condition. Therefore, when she developed complications at the beginning of the fifth month, her doctors immediately ordered her into the hospital for continuous monitoring.

After two weeks the crisis appeared to be over and Arlene wanted to go home. But her doctors wanted her to remain in the hospital so she could be monitored for the remainder of her pregnancy. Arlene suggested that she could be monitored at home, but her policy did not cover this type of home service. At this point, Arlene obtained prices of renting monitoring equipment. She also got a full accounting of her daily hospital costs, which were much higher. She then had the information she needed to negotiate with her insurance company, and home monitoring was ultimately approved.

Your Right to Receive Government Medical and Disability Benefits

Never assume that your income or your assets will prevent you from receiving public benefits. Also, don't assume that a hospital social worker will have complete information about eligibility. There are particular situations that would allow you to be eligible for benefits and although some social workers know about them, others do not.

Therefore, you should always initiate applications for any public benefits to which you think you may be entitled. These could include Workers' Compensation, Social Security Disability Insurance (if you will be unable to work for at least a year), Medicaid (if you are going to require long-term care that is not covered by your health insurance), and even home modifications through special state and municipal grants. The hospital social worker may be able to supply you with the necessary forms and assist you in filling them out. If not, you should seek other professional help. Human service agencies in your community and self-help support groups may be able to help you or they can direct you to private social workers and lawyers who specialize in helping people become eligible to receive public benefits.

If you carry any private disability coverage, either personally or through your employer, you should also submit these applications before leaving the hospital.

Rick's Story

Rick H. had been a successful salesman until, at age thirty, he became severely disabled as a result of a head injury sustained in an auto accident. Although he owned his own home, upon discharge from the hospital, he had to move into his parents' home since he could no longer live alone. Rick required ongoing rehabilitation and medical care. But because he carried private disability insurance, which guaranteed him a monthly income of $1200, he was informed by his hospital social worker that he was not eligible for Medicaid.

At the end of the first year of his recuperation, Rick had spent almost seven thousand dollars on medical care. It was only by chance, during an interview for acceptance to an out-patient rehabilitation program, that Rick and his family learned these expenses would now make him eligible to receive Medicaid for at least one year.

Summary

- Mistakes can be made even in the best hospitals. However, by EXERCISING YOUR RIGHTS AS A PATIENT you will receive much better care than you will if you are merely a passive patient. You have an obligation to yourself to be actively involved in your hospital care.
- YOU HAVE THE RIGHT to be fully informed by your doctor regarding your medical condition. Keep notes of all conversations.
- YOU HAVE THE RIGHT to know what medications you are receiving and to refuse any that you feel will be harmful.
- YOU HAVE THE RIGHT to monitor all medications, tests and procedures and your diet.
- To ensure YOUR RIGHT to adequate nursing care, your doctor can help you gain approval from your insurance company for private duty nurses.
- There are techniques you can use to develop good relationships with floor nurses and to maintain control of pain medication.

- YOU HAVE THE RIGHT to adequate medical communication even if you are unable to speak, hearing impaired or non-English speaking.
- YOU HAVE THE RIGHT to know the names, positions and functions of all hospital staff involved in your care and to request help from the hospital's patient representative.
- YOU HAVE THE RIGHT to refuse any treatment or observation that you feel is unsuitable.
- YOU HAVE THE RIGHT to considerate and respectful treatment.
- YOU HAVE THE RIGHT to appeal your discharge notice and discharge plan if you disagree with them.
- You may be able to get additional benefits through your health insurance if you are persistent and negotiate skillfully.
- The hospital social worker or outside professionals can help you to apply for any public or private benefits to which you are entitled.

SECTION THREE

YOUR RIGHT TO QUALITY CARE AFTER YOU LEAVE THE HOSPITAL

YOU HAVE THE RIGHT to expect quality medical care once you come home from the hospital. You should continue the same methods of communication and questioning that were described in Sections One and Two whenever you have contact with your doctor or other health care providers.

Your Relationship with Doctors

You can locate doctors for primary care or for second opinions through contacts with the following:

- self-help support groups;
- hospitals that specialize in treating your medical problem;
- local medical societies;
- hospital referral services.

You should thoroughly investigate the qualifications of each medical provider you are considering.

In communicating with doctors, be sure to write down the questions you need to ask and record the answers. If you are using a physician who cannot or will not communicate openly with you, you should seriously consider changing doctors.

You have a responsibility to yourself to question the purpose and ramifications of every test, medication and procedure your doctor prescribes.

Joe's Story

When Joe K. was 27, he was involved in an auto accident that left him severely brain injured. As a result, he was unable to walk, his speech was slurred and he could not perform even such basic acts as dressing himself and going to the bathroom.

After three years of intensive outpatient therapy, augmented by long hours of work each day with his home health aide and his mother, Mrs. K., Joe had significantly improved. He could now transfer from his bed to his wheelchair without help and his speech had become more intelligible. Joe was especially pleased when he could finally control his bladder, because this meant he would be allowed to participate in vocational and social programs at his rehabilitation center.

Nevertheless, Mrs. K. and the therapists at the rehabilitation center were puzzled because there were many times when Joe's jeans were wet although he reported he had recently urinated.

Mrs. K. decided to take her son to the offices of a well-known urologist and his associates. The doctor who examined Joe was the newest member of this group practice. He diagnosed Joe's condition as being due to a blockage, which caused urine to seep out after he had finished urinating. The urologist advised that surgery was the only way to correct this condition.

Mrs. K. told the social worker at the rehabilitation center about the pending operation. The social worker advised her to not only question the possible risks or side effects of the operation, but also to ask the urologist how many times he had performed this operation, how long he had practiced and whether he was board certified.

The doctor seemed surprised at these questions. When he asked Mrs. K. why she wanted this information, she replied, "Doctor, Joe is my only son and this is his only penis! I just want to make sure that he gets the best care possible."

Satisfied with the doctor's answers, Mrs. K gave permission for him to operate. She was therefore surprised to learn that the senior urologist had performed the surgery and wondered if this change was due to her questions about the younger doctor's experience and credentials.

Within a month after Joe was discharged from the hospital, he was totally cured and able to participate in the social and vocational programs at his rehabilitation center.

Monitoring Your Medications

Prescription drugs

When you are in a hospital, there is an ongoing record of all medications prescribed to you, which can be monitored by your primary physician. However, once you return home, problems related to medications can occur.

Each time a doctor prescribes a new medication for you, you must ask the following questions:

- What is the purpose of the medication?
- Are there any side effects?
- Are there special directions?

You must also give your regular doctor a list of all medications you are taking. Only in this way can a doctor be certain that she is not prescribing something that conflicts with another medication. Be sure to call your doctor immediately if you have any adverse reactions.

Never take a new prescribed medication unless your doctor is aware of every other medication you are already taking.

Grace's Story

Grace C. had been working as a volunteer in the Foster Grandparent Program for three years, giving "tender, loving care" to seriously ill children in the pediatric ward of a large hospital. When the nursing staff began to notice that Grace seemed confused at times and, occasionally, was even incontinent, the head nurse reported these symptoms to Grace's supervisor.

The supervisor visited Grace in her home, where she lived with her married daughter. The daughter had also noticed a sudden change in her mother's behavior. Upon questioning the daughter, Grace's supervisor learned that Grace had recently started going to a different doctor who had prescribed several new medications.

The supervisor urged the daughter to give a list of all Grace's medications to her new doctor and to discuss Grace's symptoms with him. With this information, the doctor quickly realized that Grace had been overmedicated and adjusted her prescriptions accordingly. Grace was soon well and able to resume her work as a Foster Grandparent.

Nonprescription drugs

You should have all your prescriptions filled by the same drugstore. Pick a pharmacist who is willing, at your request, to review all your medications prior to selling you over-the-counter remedies.

Nancy's Story

After Nancy B. was hospitalized because of blood clots in both lungs, her doctor placed her on Coumadin to thin her blood. When she left the hospital, Nancy was given a tape and a booklet about Coumadin that explained the potential danger of taking this drug in conjunction with aspirin or with certain foods and food supplements.

Nancy also realized there was a danger that she might inadvertently take some over-the-counter preparation that could interfere with the Coumadin and made a point of consulting with her druggist each time she purchased any new nonprescription remedy. In this way, she was able to manage her care so that her need for Coumadin remained consistently the same.

Patient's Rights When Receiving Home Care Services

If your hospital discharge plan states that you must receive home care services and/or treatment at an outpatient facility, YOU HAVE PATIENTS' RIGHTS similar to those you had in the hospital.   These services include the following:

- skilled nursing,
- home care aides,
- physical therapy,
- occupational therapy,
- cognitive therapy
- speech therapy,
- dialysis,
- counseling,
- and any other treatment required for your recovery.

Make sure you receive a copy of the Patient's Bill of Rights from each provider. Then read them and use them.

George's Story

George P. suffered a stroke when he was eighty which left him too weak to care for himself or to walk unaided. Because George lived alone, his doctor prescribed the services of a live-in personal care aide to assist with his care and specified that a nurse visit him weekly once he left the hospital. On the day that George returned home, the visiting nurse and a representative from the home care agency both spent time with George and his daughter, Alice, explaining the Patient's Bill of Rights as it applied to their specific services.

The doctor had also prescribed a wheelchair and a walker for George, which arrived the day before he was discharged from the hospital. Several weeks later, when Alice was filing away the invoice for her father's equipment, she noticed that, on the back, there was a Customer's Bill of Rights and Responsibilities for people leasing equipment. These rights include the right to be instructed about the function, use and maintenance of all leased equipment, and the right to select a preferred day and time for servicing the equipment. The customer's responsibilities include an agreement to maintain ordinary care of equipment and to contact the vendor about any problem with the equipment or if it is no longer needed.

Dealing with Insurance Companies

You must be as forceful in dealing with your insurance company as you were while in the hospital. There may be times when your company will try to deny payment for some treatments that you were led to believe were covered. Use every method possible to appeal this decision.

Robert's Story

When Robert H. began to recover from a spinal cord injury as a result of a car accident, he still needed skilled medical care. Because his neurologist felt he had a good chance of regaining at least some of his mobility, he recommended that Robert be transferred to a rehabilitation center that was connected to a large hospital. Before he was transferred, one of his sons and his secretary spoke to representatives of his insurance company and were assured that he was covered at 100 percent for up to a million dollars. Nevertheless, when the rehabilitation institute submitted a bill for the first six weeks of Robert's treatment, the insurance company refused to pay it because they said the policy did not cover facilities that were primarily for rehabilitation.

Robert and his family decided to fight this decision. They contacted a lawyer who discovered that another rehabilitation center had successfully overcome a similar ruling by establishing that the treatment received was medical as well as rehabilitative. The institute that was treating Robert agreed to join with him in an appeal to the health insurance company, using the same rationale. They succeeded in forcing the insurance company to reverse their decision.

Your Right to Appeal if Denied Government Benefits

YOU HAVE THE RIGHT to appeal a denial of any government benefit for which you have applied, such as Medicaid, Worker's Compensation, Supplemental Security Income and Social Security Disability Insurance. To become informed about the appeal process, seek help from a social worker or a lawyer who specializes in this field or from a community human services agency.

Anita's Story

Anita S. was a divorced woman in her early 60's who became permanently disabled as a result of a stroke. When she was discharged from an in-patient rehabilitation hospital after two months of treatment, her discharge plan included further outpatient rehabilitation and the services of a home care aide for three hours a day. The hospital's social worker realized that her present medical insurance would not cover her for prolonged home care and rehabilitation. The social worker therefore advised Anita to apply for Medicaid and gave her the appropriate forms.

Anita filled out the forms to the best of her ability and submitted them to Medicaid. After a few weeks, she was notified that her application was denied. The notice from Medicaid indicated the steps to take for registering an appeal. Anita called her local bar association and got the name of several lawyers who specialized in disability law. With the help of one of these attorneys, Anita was able to win her appeal and thus to continue to receive the ongoing services that she required.

Your Right to Prepare an Advance Directive

Now that you are home from the hospital, you need to give serious thought to one additional right that we have not discussed before.

YOU HAVE THE RIGHT to prepare an advance directive giving details of how you want to be treated medically in the event you become so incapacitated you are unable to communicate with your family and your physician.

For many Americans, their first understanding of the value of advance directives came as a result of the deaths of Richard Nixon and Jacqueline Kennedy Onassis in the spring of 1994. Both had prepared a form of advance directive known as a living will, in which they requested that extreme measures not be taken to prolong their lives in certain terminal situations.

By law, medical facilities must advise patients of this right when they are admitted. (This information is usually given to patients in writing, along with all other admitting papers.)

However, to be of any real worth, preparing these instructions requires calm, thoughtful deliberation, which is not often possible during times of physical and emotional stress.

Before developing an advance directive, you need to talk to your doctor about treatment options for specific medical conditions and to consider how you feel about living with a serious physical or mental disability. It is equally important to discuss your decisions and your reasons for making them with the people closest to you.

If you do not prepare written instructions for your medical care, doctors and hospitals may make decisions regarding treatment that are contrary to your wishes.

Alice's Story

Although Alice O. had a wonderful relationship with her two grown daughters, she had never discussed with them her desire to donate her organs and bones for transplant upon her death. After Alice was killed in an automobile accident, doctors from a nearby hospital informed her family that the hospital needed their immediate approval to remove all of Alice's viable organs and several major bones, as per the instructions on her driver's license. However, because Alice had failed to prepare an advance directive and had not talked to her daughters about her decision, they were outraged at what they felt was a violation of their mother's body. Had Alice explained her bequest to her daughters at the time she made this decision, they would have been spared the pain and anger they were now enduring and, in all likelihood, would have acquiesced to her wishes.

There are two types of advance directives: *living wills* and *durable powers of attorney for health care* (also known as health care proxies). Which form or forms must be used and whether such directives need to be witnessed or notarized depend on each state's laws.

Living Wills

The purpose of a living will is to enable you to specify, in advance, whether or not you want to be kept alive through the use of artificial life-sustaining procedures if you become unable to convey your wishes to your family and doctor.

Without this written statement, your family has no power to authorize either the use or withholding of life-sustaining procedures.

Living wills can be applied in cases of terminal conditions in all states; in some states they are also valid in instances of permanent comas.

In preparing a living will, you should consider the following questions:

- Are you willing to be fed or given fluids artificially through a tube to your stomach or intestines or through your veins? (This procedure is known as nutrition and hydration.)

- In the event that your breathing ceases or your heart stops beating, do you wish to be given cardiopulmonary resuscitation? (This treatment includes such emergency procedures as mouth-to-mouth resuscitation, external chest compression, electric shock, insertion of a tube to open a patient's airways, injection of medication into the heart, and open-chest heart massage.) If, under certain specific conditions, you do not want this treatment, your refusal is known as a do not resuscitate (DNR) order.
- In the event that you require additional assistance to continue breathing, do you wish to be put on a respirator or ventilator?
- Do you have any reservations about taking medications, including painkillers, which might either hasten or delay your death?

Some states also permit you to issue a do not resuscitate order verbally. This must be done in the presence of two adults, one of whom must be a doctor.

You can draw up your own living will if you cannot afford the services of an attorney. However, you must use the specific forms and adhere to the restrictions that the laws of your state decree. You can obtain information about forms and restrictions for your state by contacting the following sources:

- Choice in Dying supplies information on living wills for all states through its toll-free number, (800) 989-WILL.
- You can also get these forms from your local bar association or from your state department of health.

Durable Powers of Attorney for Health Care

A durable power of attorney for health care (sometines known as a health care proxy) is a much more powerful form of advance directive than a living will.

Durable powers of attorney for health care go beyond living wills in that they can be used in any situation in which an individual is no longer able to be in charge of his own medical care, not just when artificial life-sustaining measures may be called for.

Another important difference between a durable power of attorney for health care and a living will is that the former allows you to designate, in writing, some other person to act as your agent to make all or certain treatment decisions for you if you are unable to do so. The powers of your agent should be as broad as possible and should allow the agent the right to make decisions for any situation not specifically covered in your directive.

You will probably need to consult with your doctor before determining the situations in which you will empower your agent to act on your behalf. They could include:

- if you become terminally ill;
- if you are in a coma or unconscious, with no chance of recovery;
- if you suffer brain damage or brain disease that causes you not to recognize people or speak and there is no hope you will recover;
- or, if, for any other reason, you are unable to communicate with your doctor and others, even for a brief time.

Your doctor can also help you determine which procedures you do or don't want in the event of specific medical conditions. These could include such varying treatments as blood transfusions, antibiotics, surgery and abortion. If you wish to donate your organs or other body parts for transplantation, you should also indicate this fact in your durable power of attorney for health care.

Finally, you need to discuss your decisions and why you made them not only with the person you have selected to be your health care agent but also with your family and close friends.

Some states allow hospital patients to verbally name someone to serve as their agent, provided this statement is made in the presence of a doctor and another adult. States also differ as to whether durable powers of attorney for health care are legally valid. However, regardless of the status of this document in your state, you should still write down your wishes and have this paper notarized, as it will provide your family and doctor with guidelines for your care. In addition, should it become necessary for a court to intervene in your case, a judge may give considerable weight to your preferences.

Be sure to find out if your state requires special forms for durable powers of attorney for health care and whether they need to be witnessed or notarized. This information can be obtained from your state department of health and from many hospitals and health-care organizations.

Summary

- YOU HAVE THE RIGHT to quality medical care after you return home.
- You should investigate the qualifications of all medical professionals you are considering.
- You should question the purpose and ramifications of every test, medication and procedure your doctor prescribes.
- You should monitor all prescribed medications and over-the-counter drugs.
- YOU HAVE RIGHTS, similar to those of hospital patients, for all services and treatments provided to you either in your home or as an outpatient.
- You must deal forcefully with insurance companies in order to secure coverage for treatment to which you believe you are entitled.
- YOU HAVE THE RIGHT to appeal a denial of any government benefits for which you have applied.
- YOU HAVE THE RIGHT to prepare an advance directive, i.e. a living will or durable power of attorney for health care.

CONCLUSION

The development of formal patients' bills of rights came about as a result of years of effort by the American Hospital Association, courts, lawyers, legislators, advocacy organizations and many others. And the work continues. Nevertheless . . .

Patients' rights are meaningless unless you understand them and make them work for you.

We have taken you this far in demonstrating practical, step-by-step methods for taking charge of your medical treatment. The rest is up to you. Good luck!

SAMPLE DOCUMENTS

The following pages contain samples of documents referred to in the previous sections.

HOSPITAL DISCHARGE NOTICE

Date:_____

**READ THIS LETTER CAREFULLY — IT CONCERNS
YOUR PRIVATE INSURANCE BENEFITS OR MEDICAID BENEFITS
OR IF YOU ARE UNINSURED**

Dear Patient:

Your doctor and the hospital have determined that you no longer require care in the hospital and will be ready for discharge on:

Day of Week_____ Date_____

IF YOU AGREE with this decision, you will be discharged. Be sure you have already received your written discharge plan which describes the arrangements for any future health care you need.

IF YOU DO NOT AGREE and think you are not medically ready for discharge or feel that your discharge plan will not meet your health care needs, you or your representative may request a review. Contact the review agent indicated on the attached page if you would like a review of the discharge decision.

IF YOU WOULD LIKE A REVIEW, you should immediately, but not later than noon of _____ call the telephone number checked off on the attached page.

IF YOU CANNOT REQUEST THE REVIEW YOURSELF, and you do not have a family member or friend to help you, you may ask the hospital representative at (xxx) xxx-xxxx who will request the review for you.

IF YOU REQUEST A REVIEW, THE FOLLOWING WILL HAPPEN:

1. The review agent will ask you or your representative why you or your representative think you need to stay in the hospital and also will ask your name, admission date and telephone number where you or your representative can be reached.

2. After speaking with you or your representative and your doctor and after reviewing your medical record, the review agent will make a decision which will be given to you in writing.

3. While this review is being conducted, you will not have to pay for any additional hospital days until you have received the review agent's decision.

IF THE REVIEW AGENT AGREES WITH THE DISCHARGE DECISION, you will be financially responsible for your continued stay after noon of the day after you or your representative has been notified of the review agent's decision.

IF THE REVIEW AGENT AGREES THAT YOU STILL NEED TO BE IN THE HOSPITAL: for Medicaid patients, Medicaid benefits will continue to cover your stay; for private health insurance patients, coverage for your continued stay is limited to the scope of your private health insurance policy.

NOTE: If you miss the noon deadline, you may still request a review. However, if the review agent disagrees with you, you will be financially responsible for the days of care beginning with the proposed discharge date.

If you would like a review of your hospital stay after you have been discharged, you may request a review by the review agent within thirty (30) days of the receipt of this notice or seven days after receipt of a complete bill from the hospital, which ever is later, by writing to the review agent.

I have received this notice and a list of Independent Review Agents on behalf of myself as the patient or as the representative of the patient:

Signature _____ Date_____

Relationship_____Time_____

HOSPITAL DISCHARGE PLAN

Discharge Plans For You

Discharge Plan (to be completed by physician)
Medications:

_____
_____
_____
_____

Diet (Specify type):

_____

Activitiy:
_____ Full _____
_____ Restricted _____

Return Appointment:_____Phone:_____
MD Signature: _____Date:_____
* *

Special Instructions for Your Care (to be completed by RN)

_____
_____
_____

_____ Additional written instructions given to patient/signiticant other.
RN Signature: _____Date:_____
* *

Social Service Plan (if applicable) _____

_____
Social Worker Signature:_____Date:_____
* *

Contact for Follow-Up: Name   First Visit Date   Phone
(   ) MD
(   ) Clinic
(   ) Home Care
(   ) VNS
(   ) Social Work
(   ) Other
* *

I have read and understand the above Discharge Plan and I understand it is important to
follow these instruction.

Patient/Significant Other Signature: _____Date:_____

LIVING WILL

To My Family, Doctors, and All Those Concerned with My Care

I, _____, being of sound mind, make this statement as a directive to be followed if I become unable to participate in decisions regarding my medical care.

If I should be in an incurable or irreversible mental or physical condition with no reasonable expectation of recovery, I direct my attending physician to withhold or withdraw treatment that merely prolongs my dying. I further direct that treatment be limited to measures to keep me comfortable and to relieve pain.

These directions express my legal right to refuse treatment. Therefore I expect my family, doctors, and everyone concerned with my care to regard themselves as legally and morally bound to act in accord with my wishes, and in so doing to be free of any legal liability for having followed my directions.

I especially do not want:

_____
_____
_____
_____
_____
_____

Other instructions/comments:

_____
_____
_____
_____
_____

Signed: _____ Date:_____

Witness:_____ Witness:_____

Durable Power of Attorney for Health Care
(Health Care Proxy)

(1) I, _____

hereby appoint _____
(name, home address and telephone number)

as my health care agent to make any and all health care decisions for me, except to the extent that I state otherwise. This proxy shall take effect when and if I become unable to make my own health care decisions.

(2) Optional instructions: I direct my agent to make health care decisions in accord with my wishes and limitations as stated below, or as he or she otherwise knows. (Attach additional pages if necessary.)

_____
_____
_____

(Unless your agent knows your wishes about artificial nutrition and hydration [feeding tubes], your agent will not be allowed to make decisions about artificial nutrition and hydration. See instructions on reverse for samples of language you could use.)

(3) Name of substitute or fill-in agent if the person I appoint above is unable, unwilling or unavailable to act as my health care agent.

_____
(name, home address and telephone number)

_____

(4) Unlesss I revoke it, this proxy shall remain in effect indefinitely, or until the date or conditions stated below. This proxy shall expire (specific date or conditions, if desired):

_____

(5) Signature _____
Address _____
Date _____

Statement by Witness (must be 18 or older)

I declare that the person who signed this document is personally known to me and appears to be of sound mind and acting of his or her own free will. He or she signed (or asked another to sign for him or her) this document in my presence.

Witness 1 _____
Address _____
Witness 2 _____
Address _____

RECOMMENDED READING

Annas, George J. *The Rights of Patients*, 2nd ed. Carbondale: Southern Illinois University Press, 1989.

Budish, Armond D. *Avoiding the Medicaid Trap*. New York: Henry Holt & Co., 1990.

Fox, Marion I., and Truman G. Schnabel. *It's Your Body: Know What the Doctor Ordered*. Bowie, Md.: Charles Press Publishers, 1979.

Horowitz, Lawrence C. *Taking Charge of Your Medical Fate*. New York: Random House, 1988.

Inlander, Charles B., and Eugene I. Pavalon. *Your Medical Rights*, 2nd ed. Boston: Little Brown and Co., 1990.

Inlander, Charles B., and Ed Weiner. *Take This Book to the Hospital with You*. Allentown, Penna: People's Medical Society, 1993.

Knowing Your Rights: Medicare Prospective Payment System. Washington, D.C.: AARP Health Advocacy Services Program Department, 1988.

Nash, David T. *Medical Mayhem: How to Avoid It and Get the Best Possible Care From Your Doctor and Hospital.* New York: Walker, 1985.

Robin, Eugene D. *Medical Care Can Be Dangerous to Your Health.* New York: Harper & Row, 1984.

Sabatino, Charles P. *Health Care Powers of Attorney.* Washington, D.C.: American Bar Association, 1990.

Sagov, Stanley E. *The Active Patient's Guide to Better Medical Care.* New York: David McKay Co., Inc., 1976.

Sneider, Iris. *Patient Power.* White Hall, Va.: Betterway Publications, Inc., 1986.

Stutz, David R., and Bernard Feder. *The Savvy Patient: How to Be an Active Participant in Your Medical Care.* Mt. Vernon, N.Y.: Consumers' Union, 1990.

INDEX

ABOUT THE AUTHORS

BARBARA HARDT, CSW, a clinical social worker, works with a team of neuropsychologists and re-habilitation therapists in a program serving individuals with head injuries. She has also developed a course in behavior management to teach parents and spouses how to cope with the serious behavioral problems that are common to these individuals. In addition, she is involved in developing funding and programs for this population on a state level as a member of the Head Injury Services Coordinating Council of the New York State Department of Health.

Ms. Hardt has also worked as a social worker in a program serving at-risk parents and children. She is fairly unique among social workers in that she left the field of social work for several years and had a successful career in sales and marketing. During this period of her life, she wrote articles on career strategies and taught seminars on career opportunities for women who were interested in returning to the workplace. Her decision to return to social work came as a result of having sustained and overcome a traumatic accident in 1988. She then realized that she wanted to help people who had gone through similar experiences.

With coauthor Katharine Halkin, Ms. Hardt wrote a series of columns on advocacy for individuals with disabilities, which appeared in a Long Island newspaper.

KATHARINE R. HALKIN, a freelance writer, has been an advocate on behalf of others for most of her adult life. Prior to becoming semiparalyzed as a result of a spinal cord injury in 1989, Ms. Halkin was the executive director of a not-for-profit agency that protects the legal rights of public school children and individuals with severe physical and mental disabilities. Her previous employment involved her in advocacy on behalf of low income, minority and elderly people. As part of her work, she frequently presented testimony before state and federal legislative bodies on the needs of the various populations she represented and lectured extensively throughout the New York metropolitan area.

Although her spinal cord injury caused her to retire, Ms. Halkin has continued this advocacy role through her involvement with organizations that focus on health care and the needs of the homeless and persons who are disabled.